16.75

MENOPAUSE AND ITS EFFECTS ON THE FAMILY

Daniel J. O'Neill

VERSITY
SS OF
RICA

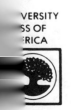

Library of Congress Catalog Card Number: **81-43827**

Acknowledgements:

Arthur F. Buckley, M.D.

Obstetrics & Gynocology

James E. Manley, M.D.

Obstetrics & Gynocology,

TABLE OF CONTENTS

CHAPTER ONE

WHAT CAUSES THE CHANGE OF LIFE?

This is the era of the liberated, well-educated,
informed woman. So we are told. When it comes to
sex, politics or how to bring up children, a lot of
magazines and books are right there with all the
answers.

But where are the answers to the hidden emotional
worries a woman experiences when inevitably confront-
ed with menopause?

"If only women understood what change of life is
all about," a medical doctor and friend once said to
me. "Too many of them are confused by superstitions
and old wives' tales. Not to mention just plain mis-
information they receive from others."

It's true. Most women, approaching, or experiencing menopause don't understand what's happening
to their own bodies. An even greater lack of information is found regarding emotional reactions to this
major change. So our primary concern will be with
these emotional troubles one may expect, along with
the more severe reactions to change of life, and how
to cope.

There are three main parts, or epochs, of a woman's life. First, puberty, where secondary sex characteristics appear, notably menstruation; second, the child-bearing years; and third, the change of life, marked by the cessation of menstruation.

Put like that it sounds simple, and it is, but each one of these important life landmarks carries with it some anxiety, some fear, and usually a lot of misunderstanding.

A young girl's first experience with menstruation often is a traumatic one, especially if proper sex education has been overlooked or avoided. Among teenage girls it can be a time of fear. Fear of pregnancy, or inability to get pregnant, or of having a retarded or otherwise imperfect baby are all too common. But in most cases youth is on the side of the girl. With its tremendous recuperative powers, problems are easier to face and easier to solve.

For some probably the best and most rewarding years are the child-bearing years. Certainly some women who have borne children will agree, on looking back, that this is so.

Where does this leave the woman who is facing the change of life? She's certainly not old. Many enjoyable and productive years lie ahead. Many of the major accomplishments of women have occurred after their menopausal period.

Unfortunately, the problems surrounding menopause are usually more intense because our modern culture is so definitely youth oriented. Advertising continually stresses the importance of looking and being young. Frustrations are bound to be experienced by attempting to be something we're not. Women have always been sensitive about growing older and our culture does everything possible to make them reject the idea.

This can become a vicious circle. No matter which way a woman turns she finds no way out of this depressing fact. This is the time she needs all the help she can get. And that is the purpose of this book.

It is only through education and understanding that a woman can take menopause in her stride and cope with it positively . . . not negatively. She has a lot of questions and she wants truths, not half truths. The healthy thing is to answer those questions. Maybe in the following list you'll find your most needed answers.

WHAT IS MENOPAUSE OR CHANGE OF LIFE?

The word menopause is derived from two Greek words meaning 'month' and 'cessation', and actually means the end of monthly periods. Therefore, in the majority of cases, it also signals the end of the childbearing period. The term change of life has the same meaning, referring to the time when your body is undergoing these changes.

AT WHAT AGE MIGHT YOU EXPECT THE ONSET OF MENOPAUSE?

It usually happens between the age of 45 and 50, although there are a few rare cases of women experiencing the 'change' before 35 years and some even after 55 years.

WHAT CAUSES THE CHANGE OF LIFE?

The inability of the ovaries to produce enough hormones. The end of ovarian activity is not always complete, which accounts for the fact that some women will continue to menstruate to some degree for several years. During this time they will also ovulate, (produce an egg also called ovum), which would account for the occasional pregnancy and subsequent 'change of life' baby.

WHAT HAPPENS TO YOU DURING MENOPAUSE?

At this point some further information on the female sexual organs is necessary in order to fully understand what happens to you during change of life, The ovaries, located on either side of the spine in the lower back of the pelvic region, produce one or more eggs (ova) every month. The wall of the uterus, located at the head of the vagina, builds up nourishing tissue in preparation for the egg (ovum). The breakdown of this tissue is what is called menstruation.

The hormone so important in menopause is also produced by the ovaries and is called estrogen. The 'change' is therefore brought about by the inability of the ovaries to produce estrogen in response to hormones secreted by another gland called the pituitary. This gland, although very small and located in the brain, is so important in its effect on all other glands that it's been called the 'master gland' of the body.

As you can see, we have a number of glands in the body which play a key role in this entire process. They secrete chemical substances called hormones directly into the blood stream and are called endocrines. The pituitary gland during the change of life becomes disturbed when the ovaries fail to respond to its secretions, which tends to affect its control over other glands. This results in a temporary imbalance existing among all the endocrine glands of the body, which could very well lead to disturbances that may involve a person's nervous system.

HOW LONG DOES CHANGE OF LIFE LAST?

The time between the first sign of menopause, usually signalled by changes in duration and intensity of your period, and the end of menopause, marked by complete cessation of the period, varies anywhere from 6 months to 3 years. Although there are a few reported cases of the 'change' lasting more than 3 years.

WHAT SYMPTOMS MAY YOU EXPECT TO EXPERIENCE?

Heading the list of some of the more common physical symptoms are 'hot flashes', and what woman hasn't heard of those? They usually involve the head and neck, but last for just a brief time. Intense sweating often accompanies these flashes. Some women report being awakened at night, finding it difficult to fall off to sleep again.

Being very excitable to ordinary situations, and feeling 'trembly', with butterflies in the stomach, are also frequent complaints. Some report shortness of breath with heart palpitations. Some complain of fatigue. Others experience dizziness. A common complaint of those prone to headaches is the increase

4

in their duration and intensity.

However, it must be understood, you may experience several of these symptoms in any combination,
or you may not experience any of them. With the ex-
ception of identical twins, in their hereditary make-
up, every woman is different. Therefore even physical symptoms are found to vary greatly from person
to person.

I am hopeful I may have answered some of your
questions. For some of you it may be enough to realize that you are suffering for a time from glandular
upset, not mental complexities. If you can think
positively, and keep as cheerful as possible during
this change in your life, your emotional troubles
will be halfway to being solved.

CHAPTER TWO

EMOTIONAL PITFALLS

Mrs. M., normally a fairly easy-going person,
found herself waking up most mornings with frustrated,
rebellious feelings. Somehow the usual habits of her
family had become maddening.

"Must you hide behind that newspaper?" She
heard her own voice rise as she eyed her husband
across the table. "Why can't you talk to me anymore?"

"So what is there to say?" Mr. M. folded his
paper with a sigh. "All right, talk. Tell me your
symptoms-all over again."

"Oh, if that's the way you feel." Mrs. M.'s
lips tightened. "Forget it." They finished breakfast in seething silence. Mr. M.'s hasty peck at
her cheek on leaving brought tears to her eyes. How
different it used to be.

Their daughter rushed through the kitchen
saying, "Hi, Mom, 'by, Mom!", and grabbed her jacket
from the hall closet. She knocked down a coat and
two sweaters in the process.

"Now see what you've done - Come back and pick
them up," commanded Mrs. M.

"Look Mom, I'm late, I'll miss the bus!"

7

Suddenly Mrs. M. felt herself losing all restraint. Words poured out of her, bitter hateful words.

"... Giving you the best years of my life! And you can't do a simple little thing for me. Of all the ungrateful..." The tirade went on and on.

"Wow - Are you ever uptight." Her daughter slammed the front door muttering, "And maybe I won't come home -ever."

Mrs. M. burst into tears. What was wrong? Was she losing her mind? Why was she so depressed, so full of self-pity? Why did she nag her husband and children? She never used to act this way. What could she do?

Later that day I walked into my waiting room to find Mrs. M. sitting there. An attractive, slightly overweight woman of 49, she sat stiffly, her gaze seemingly transfixed on a magazine picture of a young and beautiful actress.

"Pretty, isn't she, even though she can't act?" she said, apparently caught off guard and feeling the need to comment. I dismissed her remark lightly, replying that I didn't know the actress.

Mrs. M. was no sooner seated in my office than she blurted out, "Please tell me, Doctor, am I losing my mind? She swallowed frequently, wringing her hands, displaying many of the symptoms of a person in a high anxiety state. "Lately I hate myself. Yes I really hate myself."

When I asked her why, the story of the scene at the breakfast table poured out. "I can't seem to think of anyone except myself," she added. "I hurt my family with my nagging. I don't mean to - After my daughter left for school I cried and cried I felt so awful. I never used to get so upset before over such a little thing."

Reassurance that she was not losing her mind was the first priority. It took little time to win her confidence, which is so important for successful psychotherapy.

Mrs. M.'s case is not unusual. In fact her reactions are quite typical of many women during the
change. Fortunately she proved to be very receptive
to psychotherapy and consequently came to see her
problems in a different light.

First, she had many needs intensified by the
change which had to be met. Most especially she had
to feel needed by her family, and to be doing something constructive where she could enjoy a sense of
accomplishment.

Mrs. M. envied her young, attractive daughter,
although she loved her deeply. She found herself
yearning for those past years when she enjoyed youth
with its great vitality and effervescence. She felt
guilty for upsetting her husband and children, for
envying her daughter, for not (as she saw it) being
worthy of her family's love and attention.

Unfortunately, as was true of Mrs. M., many
women get on this guilt-depression anxiety merry-go-
round. As they experience depression and anxiety
from their guilt feelings, they lower their resis-
tance to stress and are therefore less able to meet
even minor problems. Mrs. M. couldn't even cope with
her daughter's untidiness. Blowing up at her daughter caused her to feel guilty, with subsequent des-
pondency and apprehension.

Another common feeling reported by many women
in the change is one of "self-pity". One woman
told me she just sat around the house all day crying.
When I asked her why she felt so dejected she hesitated.

"I don't know why," she finally admitted.
"There's no sense to it. My husband tries so hard to
be helpful."

"How about your two children?"

"Oh they're grand," was her proud reply. "Of
course they're old enough to understand. That helps."

"Any financial worries? Or other major problems in your life?"

"No." She shook her head. "That's what is so

so aggravating. I've no reason for feeling this way.
I'm really a very lucky woman." She leaned forward
anxiously. "What is wrong with me? I've got to
know."

Several sessions of psychotherapy helped her to
find the answer. She was feeling sorry for herself.
She continually dwelt on the fact that she was growing too old to enjoy life to its fullest (which she
wasn't.) That there were many things she had wanted
to do and hadn't done.

She soon realized that many wonderful years
could be hers. The change of life need not signal
the end of a full life, but rather the beginning of
an even more rewarding life, void of many of the
fears that often mar the earlier years of a woman's
existence.

Still another problem, quite prevalent at this
time, is compulsive eating. It's generally recognized as an attempt to satisfy unmet needs.

It may be complicated if the woman, which is
true of many today, is trying to recapture her
youth. One over-weight matron, dressed in a mini-
skirt and sweater more suitable for a teenager,
sought help with her problem.

It's important to understand that she, in a clin-
ical sense, was not mentally ill. She had, however,
partially regressed back to her late adolescent
period. She spent half her waking hours before a
mirror. Intense narcissism (self love), and ego-
centeredness (selfishness), characteristics of ado-
lescence, ruled her behavior. What really concerned
her was her vacillation, also typical of the adolescent period. Her changeable behavior had, and was,
costing her in both money and friends and a loss of
her daughter's respect. The nineteen year old girl
was frequently critical of her parent's dress and
actions. Her comment frequently heard was, "Oh,
Mother, really. Act your age."

As was true in this case, a woman going through
the change who had unsatisfied needs during her
growing-up stage, will have a greater chance of re-
gressing back to that period of her development.
This woman's basic problem was the fact that she had

10

to leave high school in her junior year to help support her mother.   Thus she missed out on many of the
fun years she should have had as a teen-ager.
Another case against high school drop-outs.

CHAPTER THREE

ESCAPISM: THROUGH ALCOHOL AND DRUGS

In general, women who feel unfulfilled upon reaching menopause, are certainly more likely to experience difficulty in day to day living. Therefore they seek desperately for some way of escape. And too often find it in alcohol.

Take the case of Lora, a friendly, rather untidy gregarious person. She married a man who lacked understanding and was always seeking perfection. He was unwilling to accept human frailties, particularly in his wife.

However, Lora's marriage seemed to be fairly successful, until the children were grown and had left home. Then, perhaps to fill the empty hours previously devoted to child-bearing and child-rearing, Lora discovered the afternoon cocktail party. Soon she was a frequent guest, or the hostess, at these affairs. She enjoyed herself with the group and with a few drinks.

And then one day she appeared in my office, her strained face showing the intensity of her problem. She looked too many years older than her years. Her tremoring hands were a clear indication of inner turmoil. She had passed through the menopause several years ago, but still carried the scars.

"I-I had to see you . . ." It was hard for Lora
to get the words out. "I have a-a drinking problem."
She took a deep breath then burst out, " I might as
well say it . . . I'm an alcoholic."

"Tell me," I said quietly.

"It all began, I think, during the change." Her
restless fingers twisted the strap of her purse. "At
least, that's when I started to feel tense-uneasy in
a crowd. It frightened me. I liked these people, I'd
been going to cocktail parties for years. Why should
I begin to have these strange feelings?"

However, Lora found a way to combat those uncom-
fortable feelings. An extra cocktail or two. It provided temporary relief at least. She learned that
alcohol gave her false courage, enabled her to continue the image of the gracious and fun-loving party
goer. Her dependence on cocktails grew, slowly and
insidiously.

"By and by three or four drinks weren't enough."
Lora glanced at me and away, but not before I'd seen
the misery in her heavy eyes. "Soon it was six-or
more. I found myself drinking at home alone. I'd
never done that before. Then I started having black-
outs, I'd lose whole days and not even know where they
went. And my husband . . ."

She was silent for a long moment. "He left me,
you know. A man gets tired of coming home hungry to
no supper and a wife in bed with a headache".

In a low faltering voice Lora built up the picture. Her husband was angered over frequently having
to get meals, plus numerous other domestic chores.
Soon a serious gulf developed between them. On many
occasions he was embarrassed by Lora's uninhibited
actions at the parties they attended together.

Being the type of man he was the outcome was in-
evitable. Before the completion of menopause, they
had separated, although they remained on friendly
terms.

"He couldn't take it," said Lora,"and I don't

14

blame him. Who wants to come home to someone like me?"

After several psychotherapy sessions Lora began to understand some of the reasons why she had a drinking problem. She was using alcohol as an escape from a life that had become meaningless. The children, some women's real reason for being, were gone. Her husband appeared incapable of giving her the security and aid a woman needs at this time, everything seemed rosier when viewed through a boozy haze.

Lora had been a rather passive member of Alcoholics Anonymous but after a number of psychotherapy sessions she became quite active. Understanding what led to her drinking problem, plus increased participation in A.A. has enabled her to cope with it. Two years have passed since our sessions with apparent success, for this is her longest period of sobriety for the last twelve years.

I was interested to learn that Lora made a survey of her female friends in A.A., to find out how many were past the menopause, and how many became problem drinkers during the change. Although far from scientific the results showed ten out of twelve women were past the change, eight out of these twelve giving menopause as the time when alcohol became a real problem for them.

If we examine our behavior we find we are constantly striving to accomplish certain things, such as, for instance, saving money to buy a color TV. We're always moving toward goals we set up for ourselves. But what happens when we are prevented from reaching these goals? When we have to spend that hard saved money for some emergency, some unexpected bills?

The more important the goal, the more intense will be the frustration and anxiety, if we are unable to reach it. Menopause, for some women, presents a barrier against the accomplishment of a number of goals. In some cases it is a strong maternal instinct not completely satisfied. Or again it could be a conscious or unconscious desire to be youthful. Very often it is the longing to find some unmet needs of early life.

15

However, escaping through the use of drugs or alcohol is a dangerous way, and usually leads to a cul de sac. In fact, it generally prolongs and intensifies the problem.

Escape through novels, TV viewing or movies is both acceptable and common, unless carried to the extreme. Sleeping longer is quite common at this time. Although it may be necessary, because of increased fatigue due to the stress of menopause, too often it is another way of escape.

The young generation will probably seek escape more through drugs rather than alcohol when they reach the change. Unfortunately, many are doing that now although in possession of their youth. There are a number of reasons for this, with the many pressures young people are experiencing today. Certainly, when they reach middle age and menopause, a way of coping with life's stresses will have already been established. Use of drugs may well become a major problem for women in the next few decades.

Even today a considerable number of women going through the change have become psychologically dependent upon barbiturates for sleeping, and tranquilizers for relaxing. If used with discretion, according to the direction of a physician, then they may and often do become a positive force. However, for some women, they have become a real crutch.

CHAPTER FOUR

IMAGINARY ILLNESSES

(One of my patients, a Mrs. J., related the following conversation that she had with her bridge club partners).

These four middle-aged women were enjoying their weekly afternoon of bridge and the girl talk. Lately their conversation seemed to be more uptight than it had been.

"Look at me," groaned Mrs. B. "All of a sudden I've got more wrinkles than an elephant."

"What's a few laugh lines?", retorted her partner, Mrs. T. "My figure's gone all to pot. I simply must get back on my diet," as she reached for another chocolate. "Tomorrow-".

Miss A., of indeterminate age, leaned forward and commented, "Girls- I've ordered another wig! I had to - my scalp is beginning to show through."

The fourth member, Mrs. J., herself, sighed deeply. "If you knew! I haven't felt well for a year. Headaches, palpitations, - I wake up nights and can't breathe. It's dreadful. Absolutely frightening."

17

"Oh well,. . . I suppose we've just got to put up with all this." "After all, girls, we're going through the change. And you know what THAT means."

But that's just it. Many women don't know what that means. When they find they're going through menopause they over-react. They become acutely aware of wrinkles, their graying hair, and their bulging waist-line. All perfectly ordinary signs of middle age. But all this comes at a time when a woman's threshold for stress is at an all time low. This extra burden, therefore, can be difficult to handle for some women.

Take Mrs. J., for instance. Instead of trying to accept the fact that menopause necessarily brings some discomfort, she began to dwell on her symptoms to the point where she became a more and more frequent visitor to her physician's office.

Although a number of exhaustive tests found her in good physical health she refused to accept the results.

"How could I feel this way and not have something radically wrong, Doctor?" she demanded. "I honestly do feel sick. Why, you know me - I wouldn't be here if I didn't feel so rotten."

"Very often in time of personal stress," answered the doctor, "we develop a set of physical symptoms very similar to an actual disease."

"You mean this is all in my mind?" Mrs. J. asked indignantly. "It seems impossible! Oh dear- what will I do?"

"I think psychotherapy is the answer for you." The doctor pulled his pad forward and wrote an address. "I agree with you, imaginary illness can often be as painful as real illness. However, I'm quite certain that you are in perfect physical condition."

Mrs. J. was unconvinced but made an appointment to see me the next day. I found her a charming woman, a very well-preserved fifty, modishly dressed and with a great deal of poise.

18

The first two sessions were uneventful. We
discussed minor problems and rather unimportant
matters. But the third visit was both traumatic
and fruitful.

She came in, nervous and tense, perspiration
beading her forehead. Her breathing was labored.

"I feel faint," she stated. "I'm having one
of my attacks." She gasped for air. "My heart...
I know it's my heart!"

That Mrs. J. was experiencing over-reaction to
stress was very evident from her pallor and fright.
She put her head down to her knees to combat her
faintness.

"Cup your hands over your mouth," I told her.
She eyed me in disbelief. "Go ahead, over your
nose and mouth. It will help your difficult breathing," I assured her.

To her amazement the distress lessened.

"But what is wrong with me?" she asked.

"A fairly common reaction to intense stress,"
I said, "we call it hyperventilation syndrome. To
put it simply, you panic and begin to over-breathe
and take in too much oxygen. This causes a loss of
carbon dioxide from the lungs and produces light-
headedness. Plus racing of the heart, numbness
of the hands, and other parts of the body, trem-
bling feelings and even muscle cramps."

Mrs. J.'s face lighted with hope. "What a
relief- What a wonderful relief!" She relaxed
in her chair. "You'll never know what a load
you've taken from me. I was so sure I had a bad
heart."

"That's quite understandable," I assured her.
"Now tell me, is there anything you enjoy doing,
just for fun? Or is there anything you've wanted
to do but never got around to doing?"

"Well. . .yes, there is." She hesitated then
said in a rush, "I've always thought it would be

19

fun to take up oil painting, but it seemed foolish, I don't even draw well."

"Then I prescribe that you do exactly that," I told her. "Painting is a good therapy. If you get any satisfaction from it, it's worth the attempt. Try it for a while and let me know how it works out."

Mrs. J.'s new interest worked out very well indeed. In fact, her paintings showed such promise that she enrolled in an art school. When she understood what caused her troubles, her outlook on life became so positive that her anxiety has been reduced to the level common for most people, even though she is still going through the change.

Although not an imaginary illness in the strictest sense, many people do experience what is called a psychosomatic illness. The prefix psycho means mind, and soma means body, pointing out the important role played by one's emotional state in developing certain disease conditions.

Some diseases, falling under the heading of psychosomatic illness could be peptic ulcer, hypertension and mucous colitis. In these instances actual physical damage to the body does occur. We know that depression is quite common during menopause although its duration and intensity vary greatly from woman to woman. Studies have also shown that concealed depression often manifests itself in hypochondriacal reactions, (truly imaginary illnesses,) and psychosomatic disorders.

These conditions, once developed, seldom disappear with the completion of menopause. A good many women probably spend the rest of their lives worrying about their health and possibly aggravating an imaginary illness. And the sad part is, they don't need to.

As in Mrs. J.'s case, therapy usually involves developing new interests, or activating old ones. Helping the patient to get her mind off herself is important, but it is usually best that the hobby should be one that is bolstered by an experience then it's usually worth repeating, and should be.

20

Always remember that the change of life is a natural process for all women. With understanding, the proper perspective and a large dose of common sense, it may well be the beginning of an even fuller and more enjoyable life.

Mrs. J. is so engrossed nowadays with her plans for newer and better paintings, she doesn't have time to worry about her health and the menopause.

CHAPTER FIVE

THE HUSBAND CAN HELP

If there is ever a time when a woman needs ten-
derness and sensitive awareness from her husband, it
is during menopause. She needs his understanding
throughout this period even more than she did during
pregnancy.

If the marriage fibers are strong and tight
there's really no problem. If the marriage is already rocky- you could be in trouble.

There are few more intense relationships than
that of husband and wife. You spend the major part
of your lifetime in close communication with your
mate.

The deeper experiences of life, bearing and
raising children, every day joys and heartaches, accomplishments and failures are completely shared only
by that one person.

When the boss vetoes one of his better ideas
into whose ear does the husband pour his complaints?
If their son leaves his room looking as if a tornado
had struck, and struck hard, on whose shoulder does
the wife collapse when he arrives home from the long
hard day at the office? Right. And this is good.

23

It means the married couple have a mutual love and respect for each other and trust. They share each other's woes as well as happiness.

On the other hand, where the relationship is strained, and many are, the years of menopause can be sadly lacking in marital harmony.

And in this trying time for the wife, it is the husband who should try to strengthen the relationship. Of necessity he will be a very important source of ventilation for his wife's emotions during the change. If any sacrifice is required then he must be prepared to make it. In the long run, if he is considerate and helpful, he will most certainly benefit.

Sometimes this can be difficult, especially if the wife is more dominant. Quite early in marriage John had relinquished much of his role as father and head of the family to Betty. This resulted in a slightly matriarchial (mother led) home. Over the years she accepted more and more responsibility, and increasingly made more decisions.

When I first met Betty her emotional tension centered on her family, mainly on her youngest son. A typically rebellious adolescent, he seldom wrote home from college, and then usually to ask for money. While home on vacation, his mother complained, he was a 'star boarder who's late for meals and leaves his room a shambles.'

Betty had repeatedly asked her husband to speak to his son, but John was too busy or had some excuse for not supporting Betty. As our sessions went on, one fact grew very apparent. The husband and wife relationship was not and never had been good, but only marginal.

True, part of the problem was created by Betty, but, of course, had John been a man of sterner metal, Betty might not have been forced into the more dominant role. Basically, women want the male partner to assume leadership. So Betty was in a predicament.

By taking over and making most of the decisions, when the time came that she needed support from

John she found that he had learned to rely on her.

By its very nature decision making and subsequent responsibility is nerve tensing. At this point it was necessary to bring the husband for psychotherapy and to assist both of them in changing their roles back to where they both provided support for one another.

John was agreeable and obviously wanted to help. Unfortunately, in his zeal, he went a bit over-board particularly in assisting Betty's decision-making. This aggravated her feelings of inferiority which are commonly experienced by women during the change. To be successful John had to be subtle and very gradually assume this new role. Another mistake he made was being too patronizing, which in part was an over reaction to his guilt feelings. This only tended to encourage Betty's already flourishing self-pity.

When John finally understood that he should become more sensitive to Betty's need to be reassured that she hadn't lost any of her feminine appeal, that she still looked attractive and dressed smartly, that she was still a woman, matters began to straighten out.

Betty showed a marked improvement in our next session. "For the first time in years John and I can sit down together and talk to each other," she said happily. "He's urging me to take up a hobby, and best of all, he's really talking to our son as a father should."

Betty, too, had undergone a little soul-searching. She had believed John's behavior meant he was indifferent and unfeeling. However his position had been one of avoidance because of fear of doing the wrong thing. His own self-concept (opinion of himself) was poor. As a result of abdicating most of the responsibility to Betty he had lost a lot of his confidence. But now both of them understood how important each was to the other.

On the other hand, there were Cathy and Jim. Although Cathy was undergoing problems in menopause, Jim did all the talking. Considering it was the first meeting his discussion of his wife's problems, in great depth, caused her obvious embarrassment. This kind of overexposure can result in an insurmountable barrier to further counseling.

Here there was absolutely no question, Jim was the dominant one in this marriage. Not only was he extremely demanding, he was a perfectionist. Cathy wasn't allowed to put his shirts in his bureau— they had to be in just a certain place and order. Also it was obvious that he looked with disdain upon any personal weakness of frailty.

Marriage had become one long ego-shattering disillusionment for Cathy. For years she had tried to come up to her husband's expectations, with little success. And now she was trying to cope with the change.

Jim had many complaints, and all of them selfish. Cathy wasn't doing her job. Several times in the past month he'd come home to find no dinner and Cathy lying on the couch. And when he merely spoke to her about it she flew to pieces-just because he told her not to be so lazy! The least little thing made her cry. To top it off, there was the matter of her sexual coldness after these arguments. Oh yes, Jim was certainly suffering through Cathy's menopause.

Unfortunately, this lack of understanding by Jim was causing a real gulf to develop between them. It's a sad commentary on life, when one considers the countless numbers of married couples who allow relatively minor problems to snowball into irreconcilable separations.

After several sessions communication between Jim and Cathy did improve. Jim couldn't be expected to change his life style, or personality, but he did become more sensitive to the trials of Cathy during menopause.

We are not islands unto ourselves, but small parts of this sea of humanity. It's natural for us to turn to those closest to us when we are troubled. For most women in menopause this is the husband.

CHAPTER SIX

DO YOUR CHILDREN KNOW?

How many times do we as parents try to shield
or protect our children from the harsh realities of
life. A great many psychiatrists and psychologists
would agree that too early an exposure to some of the
more stressful aspects of living may cause emotional
trauma with unhealthy consequences. An acquaintance
of mine believed that fantasy and other forms of un-
reality had no place in the life of a child. Santa
Claus, the Easter Bunny and other childhood fantasies
were restricted from the very real world of his children. Certainly they were required to face at a very
early age many of the difficulties that beset man.
Unfortunately, major adjustment problems have been
experienced by all of his children.

One problem facing mothers experiencing menopause is do you tell your children about the "change
of life" or do you keep it from them. In some ways
it presents the same difficulties as does sex education. How much information do you provide and at
what age? However, the majority of women at this
stage of their lives have children that are in ado-
lescence or are young adults. But if pre-school or
pre-adolescent youngsters are involved then some
care must be taken in presenting information rele-
vant to this problem.

One mother whose youngest child was a boy nine

years old had her husband explain to his son that "mommy is having some change occur in her body. It's not something you can see but it's perfectly normal, and there's nothing to worry about, in fact all women around mommy's age experience this. But sometimes mommy is upset easily because of these changes." Again we must not fail to recognize individual differences. As mentioned previously the majority of women pass through the climacteric without serious difficulty. However, even milder changes in a mother's personality may be disruptive to her children. Also the children can be expected to react differently according to their sex, age, relationship with mother, emotional make up and social relationships.

It would seem reasonable to assume that children of pre-school age being in the important formative years would psychologically suffer most in the menopausal home. The mother-child relationship is of paramount importance in personality development. What happens if the mother's relationship to her child is one of vacillation, instability, and rejection as a result of menopause? Many experience a variety of feelings from guilt and depression to considerable insecurity and, above all, a poor self-concept. (how he sees himself and how he sees his environment in relation to himself.)

The basic course of healthy self-development is usually described in terms of eight psychological stages of development. The first is the sense of trust, which normally emerges during the first year of life. Most infants have little trouble developing a sense of trust because their needs at this age are nearly always satisfied. However, the next stage-the sense of autonomy- may pose some real problems. This begins at twelve or fifteen months until four or five years old. At this stage the child begins to assert his own individuality. Parents, particularly the mother, should be consistent in both what they allow and forbid him to do.

The above two stages plus the sense of initiative are all formed during early childhood and are basic to successful development at later stages. It is conceivable that many personality disorders have their origins in this early period. Fortunately, a few women have "change of life" babies and the majority of these are not severely affected.

Certainly many more adolescents have mothers in menopause and therefore are more likely to face the problems of trying to maintain a good mother-child relationship. Unfortunately, the adolescent's personality often parallels the mother's in being egocentric, vacillating and often irrational. However, for the adolescent, this behavior is expected but not for a mature, slightly past middle age woman. This probably contributes greatly to many of the personality clashes between mother and adolescent.

Next to my desk sat a young college student of 19. He was visibly nervous, fidgeting and constantly rolling a pencil back and forth between his fingers. This was our second session and it appeared many more would be required in order to win the confidence of this reticent and anxious young man.

A sudden emotional outburst of deep sobbing occurred, and I realized that this release signaled the beginning of a valuable psychotherapeutic session. The words flowed out as if under great pressure resulting from months or even years of tension building.

As is true in the vast majority of cases, Bill had a multitude of problems. Being around an age when his sex drive is most intense and constantly stimulated by the suggestive dress of coeds (miniskirts, etc.) plus emphasis on sex by our mass media, rather intense sex frustration was one of his problems.

Academically, his work was fair, although he studied long hours ostensibly requiring a more than average effort on his part.

Sex and the pressure of college academic work are problems faced by scores of our young people. Fortunately, the majority are able to resolve these problems with little or no professional help.

The majority of adults, be they parents or not, are aware of all this. But have we fully considered the effect on a young man or woman of his mother's changing personality due to menopause? The young

29

man seated next to my desk needed professional help with this problem above all others. His living at home and commuting to school rather than living in residence on campus did not help. More and more students are able to live at home while in college, due to the close proximity of institutions of higher learning such as community colleges. The financial benefits to parents are considerable, but it may be at some cost.

Bill fully talked about the difficult and very tense home environment resulting from his mother's vascillating and irrational behavior. To further intensify the problem, Bill came from a matriarchial home. It can be very disruptive to the family when the one individual who is the stabilizing and guiding force in the home is undergoing changes in personality.

Bill's problem was partially resolved by leaving home. He moved nearer the campus sharing an apartment with two other students. But even more important was Bill's lack of understanding of the "change of life." Although he had fourteen years of formal education he confessed complete ignorance of the subject. Several in depth discussions provided the knowledge of menopause a young man in his position needed. He later stated "many times I unnecessarily antagonized my mother, but I certainly wouldn't if I had known. Now I'm more tolerant and believe me we're getting along okay."

An additional problem faced by menopausal mothers with teenage children is adolescent rebellion. All adolescents experience this to some degree. We recognize this as a natural and even necessary part of their psychological development. If they are ever to become full-fledged adults they must gradually challenge the parental authority exercised over them. Fortunately, most young people do this without undue stress or alienation of parents. But this emancipation to adult status can provide an additional stress to the mother whose threshold for stress may already be lowered by the change.

A lack of knowledge and a lack of understanding go hand in hand. Parents with this common problem have both a right and a responsibility to enlighten their children on the subject. Instead of being

30

critical of their thoughtlessness and lack of concern, give them an opportunity to help, by first in-
forming them of the change of life.

CHAPTER SEVEN

ALONE AND EXPERIENCING THE CHANGE

So far most of our discussion has been concerned with the wife and husband relationship. What of the many other women, the unmarried, the widowed, the divorced?

Margaret was single. Since her father died when she was a child, she and her mother were very close. While her mother was alive Margaret's life was full and satisfying. She had learned to rely on her mother for all her social needs.

Then the mother died suddenly, and Margaret's sheltered life collapsed. She had devoted so much of her time, outside of her job to her mother, that she had lost contact with other people. Now she was left with long, empty nights and weekends.

To add to her misery, Margaret was going through the change. Her depression and loneliness became overwhelming. She suffered from a deep sense of rejection.

So intense was her need for friendly contacts she began to spend weekends at a nearby hotel. She couldn't bear to stay in her desolate house. This didn't help too much because her mother had been a strong believer that thrift was a virtue. And so, on top of everything, she felt extremely guilty

33

about the expensive weekends.

Fortunately Margaret wanted to do something about the dilemma she found herself in. She didn't want to waste any more of her life being lonely, depressed, bored and just generally unhappy. And so she came to me.

Being a sensible woman she acted on the suggestions I gave her. Some very dramatic and positive changes occurred. She sold her house and bought a condominium where social contact was assured. Although selling one's home is not often advised, in her case it did help. She joined several organizations in which she'd always been interested. She made a lot of new friends of different ages and backgrounds. Then she started to travel during vacations to places she'd always wanted to go.

During our last session she admitted, "I never realized how much joy one could find in life!"

Jane was a widow of one year. Most women face a hard period after the loss of a husband. For Jane it was exceptionally unbearable. She and her husband had had a very happy marriage.

"I just can't put into words the loneliness I feel," she told me. "I'm...hollow. And my son is grown now. When I think of his leaving home-I get frightened."

Jane hadn't worked outside her home since her marriage. She also hadn't developed any special skills that she could use now. Her whole life for the past twenty-two years had centered on her family and home. She had been a completely contented and domestic housewife. Suddenly her world was shattered. And at the same time she was going through menopause.

The problem now was to guide her in putting the pieces back together to form a new life. Psychological testing uncovered latent talents and interests she needed to develop. Psychotherapy helped guide her in resolving emotional barriers to the accomplishments of these goals. She's now completing her senior year of college and looking forward eagerly to a career in social work. This is an area for which she'd always had a great interest.

Needless to say, her outlook on life is good, and her major problems are solved. She is looking forward with much anticipation to becoming a grandmother. When her son married, instead of bemoaning the loss of her son she found she had gained a daughter. Her strong positive attitude is the result of her successful adjustment to leading a new and rewarding life.

Karen's case was a little different. She was divorced. She wasn't bereft in the same way as Jane, but her self-concept had been quite badly damaged.

"I never realized it was going to be so hard," she confessed, her face sad and drawn. "It wasn't easy, knowing my husband found another woman to share his life with. But now-I'm neither a wife, or a whole woman. I can't see any future...."

"You can pick up the pieces," I told her. "Make a new life for yourself."

"How can I?" she demanded. "When the change is over I won't be feminine-I won't have any more sex appeal. I'll be a shell."

"Make as many new friends as possible," I advised her. "And build up your self-confidence. It can be done, although it will be hard, especially at first. But you must make the effort. Menopause is NOT the end of the world for you."

"Well...I'll try," she said doubtfully, "but I don't know if I can."

"Always remember there are many, many women in the same boat," I said. "Give it a try anyhow."

Karen proved to be a stronger person than she knew. She did try- and succeeded. Perhaps her new life isn't as satisfying as her previous state, but today she's a fairly happy, busy person.

Unmarried women, or those without husbands as a result of death or divorce, need someone to confide in. Although it's doubtful that a relative or friend can be as close as a husband, still many basic emotional needs can be met by such a person. Actually most women in this situation do have such relationships. It is most important to keep these friendships and make new ones while going through the change.

However don't limit yourself by spending all your time with other women who, like yourself, are experiencing, approaching or are just past the change. It's great to have friends who can sympathize, but it can be overdone. And don't isolate yourself from people. This is bound to have a devastating affect on your ego. The woman who does restricts herself to a myopic vision of her environment. Get out there and have fun, even if you don't feel like it.

Develop new interests, broaden your horizon. You may be surprised to find this period of your life one of the most satisfying and fulfilling. Isabella Taves, in her current book, "Women Alone", considers happiness not a goal but rather "It is a by-product that comes and goes..." How often you find happiness and how long you hold on· to it, depends on you.

If, like Margaret, Jane and Karen you learn to cope with the problems of menopause, keep active and re-pattern your social life, this part of your life will hold no terrors. It may be a more mature contentment, but then you are a more mature person. You will be able to take anything, including menopause, in your stride.

CHAPTER EIGHT

THE ANTICIPATORY SYNDROME

An article in Reader's Digest caught my attention: it was titled "My Journey Into Darkness." The author was a woman who had developed a serious mental illness during and because of menopause. She discussed her terrible experiences with some vivid details that would scare many women facing the change into a state of near shock. Certainly for years the subject was seldom discussed. However, when it was it often resembled the horror stories told around a campfire by the young scouts to see who could frighten the most people. Consequently, many misconceptions and many unnecessary fears surround this very normal period of a woman's life.

With approaching middle age some anxiety and apprehension is common particularly in our youth oriented society. It's unfortunate that many people find this a time of life when feelings of regret begin to be felt. There also appears to be a greater tendency to fall victim to fear laden tales with subsequent problems. Many women prior to menopause are traumatized by the often repeated and often grossly exaggerated stories of the few who did experience real difficulty at this time.

It certainly can lead to anxiety which is a state of uneasiness and foreboding with the individual being apprehensive of impending disaster. In a number of cases it has been so intense that it brought on several of the symptoms of menopause. Some women in their middle or late thirties (not that small number that experience the change early) have even reported hot flashes, nervous excitability and irregular periods. More often than not they blame an early menopause for their problems, although in a few instances a biological cause is found. In most cases it's the result of anxiety.

Dr. Coleman in his book on personality states, "Fear may exaggerate the severity of the problem and generate an attitude of apprehension which makes it all but impossible to follow any course of action." And it may also create problems where none exist.

Barbara was referred to me by her physician after complaining of symptoms characteristic of the "change of life." However, it was determined that she was probably many years from this experience. Nevertheless, she did require help with her anxiety state. It came as no surprise when she arrived a half hour late for her first appointment. She had never before been to a psychiatrist or psychologist and for days had been living in fear of our first session.

Barbara was a slim attractive woman whose outward appearance was one of great charm and self-confidence. She made a great effort trying to convince me that she didn't have a problem. Encouraged to talk, the conversation soon centered on her mother and father. She lived with both her parents and had a surprisingly good relationship with them. Although she had never married this did not prevent her from enjoying a very full social life. Being a teacher she had time to travel summers and had vacationed in many parts of the world. A large circle of friends, a good home environment and a job that provided great satisfaction did not prevent her from being a victim of intense anxiety.

Being very close to her mother she was still a bit naive in her accepting as fact anything her mother said. Her mother's circle of friends were all

post menopausal. Therefore, it was understandable
that guests at the afternoon cocktail party frequently discussed as a topic of common interest, the
change of life. And Barbara's mother always related
to her in great detail all the conversation, etc.,
that transpired. Fear of menopause had undoubtedly
started at an early age and was constantly being re-
inforced. As she passed into middle age she felt
the narrowing of time; she was getting closer to
that epoch in life upon which she looked with such
fear. Anxiety continued to build up to a point
where it actually affected her biological processes.
As were previously mentioned in Chapter 4, Imaginary
Illnesses, the mind and nervous system can alter a
number of physical reactions. Some women have had
the experience of missing their period when under
intense emotional stress.

In Barbara's case the symptoms of menopause
were very well known. With her increasing anxiety
she partially thought herself into a psychological
state of menopause. However, her symptoms were far
more severe (even somewhat bizarre) than is experienced by most women at this time of life. This
very intense negative anticipation of the change of
life brought on this pattern of behavior (syndrome).
A dramatic and positive change occurred in Barbara's
personality as she gained insight into her dilemma.
In a few months she was enjoying life without this
intense fear and minus the characteristic symptoms
of menopause.

A positive preparation for menopause should
start early. If a woman is acceptant of her changing
roles, then the approach to the change and the actual
transition later should present little or no problems. This really begins prior to puberty when a
girl is encouraged to accept the new role of a young
lady. Marriage, child bearing and rearing all con-
stitute new roles and the ease with which she accepts
these is certainly an indication of how she'll
accept the change of life.

CHAPTER NINE

SHOULD YOUR SEX LIFE CHANGE
WITH THE CHANGE?

To listen to the young generation you'd think
they invented sex, or that it belongs to them exclu-
sively. Since they honestly feel that anyone over
thirty is utterly comatose, no doubt the suggestion
that middleaged married couples can still enjoy sex,
would be an unbelievable statement.

Lately teen-agers and young adults have come under rather close scrutiny by many of the older mem-
bers of society for their liberal views toward sexual
freedom and expression. The advertising industry and
mass media in general have attempted to capitalize on
this very important drive.

Little or no attempt has been made to communi-
cate the continued importance sex plays in the lives
of those in middle or older years.

Many studies have been made concerning the role
of sex in the lives of people, the best known perhaps
being the Kinsey, Masters-Johnson, and Isaac Rubin
Reports, but it is still not clearly understood. One

myth, borne out by some philosopher's comment, "Isn't it too bad that youth is wasted on the young?", is that the sex drive automatically declines with age. When a man challenges this with continued virility into his older years, he's labeled a 'dirty old man.' This also goes for older women who still function as complete, whole human beings.

Investigations by behavioral scientists into sexual behavior, encountered many problems. Many strong emotions are conjured up in an individual when faced with questions dealing with his sex life. Teenagers have been reluctant to participate for fear of exposure. But in the case of older people, nobody cares and nobody asks.

What are the facts concerning sex indulgence after the change? First, your erotic drive is culturally determined, and therefore not directly dependent on the presence, or absence, of sex hormones. Too many people are inclined to feel that sexual intercourse is now unnecessary because reproduction is no longer possible.

If you have been brought up to believe that the main purpose of sex is to produce children, and that the drive only operates to fulfill this function, then your continued pleasure in your sex life is doubtful. For many women, and quite a few men as well, the pleasurable aspects of sex have never been realized. However it's never too late, whether the couple is young, middle-aged or well past the change.

A Mr. and Mrs. B. were referred to me by their physician. Both were in their late fifties, but she was younger in appearance. Four years had passed since her menopause, but she was left with a problem. Psychotherapy sessions were held both individually and together.

Mrs. B. was quite relaxed in therapy, quickly relating all the events of her difficulty. Prior to menopause she enjoyed a good sex life. There was seldom any delay in reaching a climax.

"Ed is... well, for me, the ideal mate," she said. "Oh, we have our battles now and then. Who doesn't? But we enjoy each other. And not just in bed." She shook her head and sighed. "However that's our problem now. And it's all my fault."

It began with the onset of menopause. Instead of being satisfied with intercourse two or three times a week, Mrs. B. would wake her husband in the morning, even though they'd had a sexually satisfying night. She became most aggressive which was contrary to her very feminine nature.

"I've always enjoyed it," she said candidly, "but up to now I've never been the one to start anything. Poor Ed, he just can't take it-and I just can't seem to help myself!"

A private session with Mr. B. disclosed that at first he was pleased with his wife's ardor which enhanced his male ego. But it was short-lived. Soon he started complaining because she was demanding just too much. It had reached the point where his male ego was taking a beating.

Mrs. B. was relieved to learn she'd spoken more truly than she knew. She couldn't help her surging sex urge. Sub-consciously she felt that the end of menstruation meant the end of pleasure in sexual intimacy. Also her days of being able to conceive were drawing to a close. Unconsciously she wanted to cram into those last few months all the sexual love of a lifetime.

Then the whole picture began to change, around the middle of Mrs. B.'s menopause. She had no more urges. Mr. B. could sleep all morning, and all night for that matter. From being sexually insatiable Mrs. B. became passive, unless Mr. B. made strong demands.

Naturally this was difficult for him to understand or adjust to. Guilt feelings developed between them. The situation became so strained they even had separate bedrooms.

After more consultations they began to see the problem from a different vantage point. They were more aware of the causes and more sensitive to the needs of the other. A year has now passed since their last session, and from all appearances things are going well with them.

Mrs. D. was a short, rather stocky woman of near-

43

ly fifty. Although in menopause she had few of the usual symptoms, she worked full time and ran the house for her two adolescent children and husband. Her concern was her lack of sex drive. She avoided her husband's advances. A coolness began to develop between them.

She tried to assure him she still loved him, but he began to have doubts. Only one session was required to help Mrs. D. She worked eight hours a day, then came home to all the household tasks. Naturally she found herself "dragging to bed", so worn out she fell asleep almost immediately. It's a medical fact that women react to fatigue by losing their sex drive and sexual interest. Mrs. D. didn't realize this.

Prior to menopause she had the energy to work full time and still meet her husband's needs. Now she was physically unable to fill all her roles. Changing her schedule, with more time for rest and relaxation, solved her problem.

CHAPTER TEN

NUTRITION CAN MAKE THE DIFFERENCE

Barbara was referred by her physician for help
with problems associated with the change of life. Although only 49 years old, she looked much older than
her years. Apparently life had not been kind to her.
Her features were good but unfortunately were framed
in dry, stringy hair, dull lifeless appearing eyes,
and unnecessary wrinkles. In our initial discussion
she made reference to her physician's comments about
the need to follow certain rules of good health, the
need for sleep, fresh air and sunshine, exercise and
a good balanced diet.

"I'm not doing anything different from what I've
always done. I get plenty of sleep and with two teenage sons and a husband to cook for, do the laundry
for, plus the housework I get plenty of exercise.
Whenever I have the time I get outdoors even in the
winter when many of my friends don't venture from
their houses."

She continued to mention that she often skipped
breakfast but had one or two cups of black coffee before lunch. Lunch often consisted of a sandwich and

45

another cup of black coffee. Dinner in the evening was usually in the seven course category and a gourmet's delight. Although often too nervous to eat much during the day, Barbara reported that she relaxed toward evening with the help of a cocktail or two. One does not have to be a nutritionist to see the harmful effect of such a diet. Numerous cups of stimulating coffee can make anyone edgy and certainly isn't going to be helpful to a woman in menopause. Many experts in nutrition feel that breakfast is the most important meal. It's felt that the energy you need for a lot of the day's work comes from breakfast.

Barbara was having a problem with her weight. Certainly eating a large,calorie loaded meal a few hours before bedtime can contribute to a weight gain. Having the same intake of food around noon will not present the same problem for calories taken in are utilized in the day's activities. If it's true that "you are what you eat" then Barbara's change-of-life problems were greatly aggravated by her diet.

Many women drink little or no milk by the time they reach middle age. Milk is a good source of Vitamin D and calcium and there's probably a greater need for these during menopause than at any other time. Women with many of the symptoms of the "change", hot flashes, nervousness, irritability, and depression have shown marked improvement when given Vitamin D and calcium.

Vitamin E has often been referred to as the anti-sterility vitamin. It's found in whole wheat, wheat germ, etc. A lot of the over-processed white bread we eat today is deficient in this vitamin. The possibility of a large number of our population being deficient in this vitamin can't be dismissed. A four year study at the College of Physicians and Surgeons of Columbia University utilized hundreds of animals past their menopause to see whether the aging process was in any way affected by Vitamin E. Results showed that the less Vitamin E given, the higher the number of sick animals. When Vitamin E was adequate in the diet of these animals, it had a striking effect on prolonging their youth. A diet deficient in this vitamin also resulted in a loss of sex interest for both sexes to the point where the animals would not mate.

46

From the results of this research it appears that Vitamin E plays a role in the production of normal sex hormones.

Anemia has long been recognized as a common problem among women. Irregular menstruation during the "change" plus an inadequate diet can certainly cause this iron deficiency. Foods containing the B vitamins and proteins will supply this needed iron. It may be more than coincidence that many of the symptoms of menopause are the same for anemia, depression, needless fatigue and mental confusion.

Barbara not only complained of all of these symptoms but also stated "I've been so forgetful lately that I really wonder if I'm getting senile prematurely or just losing my mind." Her problems were only temporary for in a few months she reported feeling "better than I've felt in years." Psychotherapy had helped but in this case some basic health guidance in nutrition really made the difference.

NUTRITIONAL NEEDS TO LOOK AND FEEL GOOD

NUTRIENT	WHAT IT DOES FOR YOU	SOME GOOD SOURCES
Protein	Builds body tissues such as muscles and blood; helps to prevent premature wrinkling of skin	Cheese, milk, meat, fish, poultry, eggs
Carbohydrates	Supplier of energy; gives you the "get-up and go" that you need	Sugars and Starch
Fats	Stored fat just below the skin contributes to the smoothness of the skin itself	Butter, lard, fat on meat
Minerals: Calcium and Phosphorus	Necessary for good teeth and bones; also important for proper functioning nervous system	Milk and cheese, lean meat, wheat breads, fish, eggs, liver
Iodine	Regulates metabolism and growth	Iodized salts and sea foods
Iron and Copper	Formation of red blood cells (hemoglobin); necessary to help you feel good	Liver, lean meat, eggs, whole or enriched grain, bread or cereals, poultry, fish

48

Vitamins:		
A	Contributes to healthy skin; helps in maintaining resistance to infection, good for your eyes.	Fish, liver, whole milk, egg yolk, butter, deep yellow and leafy vegetables
B_1 (Thiamine)	Good for healthy nerves and good digestion	Whole and enriched grain products, muscle meat, beans, liver, egg yolk, oysters
Vitamin B_2 (Riboflavin)	Good for skin around nose and for lips and tongue	Milk, cheese, liver, egg yolk, lean meat, whole and enriched grain breads and cereals, leafy vegetables
Niacin	Good for healthy nerves, skin and mucous membranes	Liver, yeast, lean meat, kidney, milk, whole and enriched grain, salmon and leafy vegetables
Vitamin C (Ascorbic Acid)	Necessary for good teeth, bones, blood vessels, helps resistance to infections, particularly the common cold	Citrus fruits, turnips, tomatoes, cabbage
Vitamin D	Important in normal bone formation and maintenance and repair; good for healthy nerves	Vitamin D milk, fish-liver oil, salmon
Vitamin E	Necessary for maintenance of sex drive; food for nervous system	Muscle meat, nuts, whole grain, wheat-germ and cotton seed oil

49

CHAPTER ELEVEN

DO MEN EXPERIENCE THE CHANGE?

Do men experience the change? The answer to this question is a definite NO. But neither do men have babies or experience a monthly period. The production of hormones in men namely androgen gradually declines over most of their adult lives, but there is no particular time when their bodies go through as profound a biological transition as do women. So why do some men experience symptoms that closely resemble those of women in menopause?

There are a number of possible answers to this question. First it may be that in our attempt to achieve sexual equality we've failed to recognize some fundamental differences between the sexes. Male and female sex roles have moved from their traditional position where men were considered more scientific, logical and competitive and women more romantic, affectionate and emotional to one which allows if not encourages a broader range of experience. Overlapping sex roles may be responsible for behavior labeled androgynous which refers to individuals having both masculine and feminine traits. Unisex clothes and media hype have contributed to the concept of sameness between the sexes. Over zealous feminists have tried to sell the idea of the male menopause as a way of pointing out that there's no real differences between the sexes. More impressionable men in expecting a menopause may actually experience its symptoms.

Another possibility is the overly empathic husband who may have experienced labor pains and even morning sickness when his wife was pregnant. Now she's in menopause and he's sharing that too.

However I believe the following case of Glenn better explains why some men do experience symptoms similar to those of women in menopause.

Glenn, a 48 year old office manager, complained of a pounding heart beat, breathlessness, undue sweating, tightness in the chest, sweaty palms, weakness, cramps, difficulty sleeping, fatigue, tension headache and sexual problems. After a complete physical exam he was diagnosed as experiencing nothing more than anxiety. Anxiety is not a disease but merely a vague fear accompanied by a feeling of uneasiness.

Glenn's physician referred him to me. Several sessions of psychotherapy brought to the surface the causes of his anxiety. What he'd mistakenly thought was male menopause was a condition brought on by business and financial problems. A 'snowball' effect occurred because the high level of stress he was experiencing curbed his sexual interest. He was beginning to believe he was all "washed up" sexually because of a few instances of impotence. Unfortunately his attitude toward sex was actually causing the very thing he feared. Sex researchers have shown that the vast majority of potency problems are psychological in nature with fear or anticipation of failure or underlying depression being the most common.

To add to Glenn's anxiety is the fact that many men go through an unsettling period usually between the ages of 40 to 50. This "mid'life" crisis is characterized by self-doubt, depression, sudden career changes, sexual problems, extramarital affairs and divorce.

A number of researchers have pointed at the

middle and upper class professional as the most vulnerable. High expectations, coupled with a desire to get the most out of life, may now lead to disillusionment and questions about what's really been accomplished. Complicating this is our culture's worship of youth and sex appeal.

Graying and thinning hair, receding hair line, balding, wrinkles, sagging eyelids and jaw, developing a "pot" certainly conjure up feelings of "heading downhill".

But recognizing that you're not alone that many other men also are faced with these challenges can help. A constructive approach is to take inventory of your past accomplishments. Be realistic of your appraisal of what you've done and also what you might do in the future.

Glenn, through greater insight into his problems, was able to constructively solve them. His improved relationship with his wife paralleled reduction in his anxiety level and a movement out of the mid-life crisis.

CHAPTER TWELVE

PROS AND CONS OF ESTROGEN REPLACEMENT THERAPY

Mrs. K. was a classic example of a woman going "cold turkey" through menopause. She was a young looking 46 and very attractive. She was happily married and had three children, two teenagers were living at home and one son was in the service. I'd describe her as emotionally healthy. Her husband and I were her only confidants during this time. To her children and others she kept up a very positive image and always had a smile. Even her physician was told only about her general physical symptoms. She was afraid he'd prescribe medication if he knew that there were many days that life was only an existence due to an intense hormone imbalance.

The usual sign of irregularity in her monthly period was diagnosed by her gynecologist as premenopausal in nature. As her periods became farther apart she first noticed a thumping type feeling on infrequent occasions which she later described as someone drumming in her chest. The next significant symptom were flashes which woke her every night and about 6 a.m. each morning. This was particularly difficult for Mrs. K. as she had to get up at 7 a.m. to go to work.

Sometimes during the intense flashes and flushes she would remain very quiet and not expend energy until they passed. They were sometimes accompanied by a feeling of someone injecting a hot fluid into her head. She reported the right side of her forehead perspiring more than the left side and speculated as to whether her left handedness was responsible. Accompanying feelings of slight cramping and backache were so similar to her monthly period that she referred to it as her "pseudoperiod".

There was normal bladder functioning during the day but her sleep was disturbed by having to void during the night. Feelings of weakness sometimes occurred but then would pass quickly. She had never experienced depression before but now her mood swings were mercurial. Sometimes she was very hopeful of future plans but other times feelings of hopelessness and despair of getting old took over. During this time a teenage child started causing problems which aggravated her condition.

Her figure started changing to what she called a "jello body" around the waistline. Occasionally her abdomen would extend similar to a woman 6 months pregnant, then it would disappear and her youthful figure would return. Fluid retention, not fat, was the cause. An unusual symptom involved her olfactory senses. She reported sensing odd odors such as machine oil or at times a sweet flower odor even after showering. Her husband never detected this, however.

When traveling to Georgia in the spring Mrs. K. suffered from the heat so intensely that she had to be revived on one occasion. Women may be more effected by high atmospheric temperature during the change of life.

Professionally trained and employed she was always very competent in her work. But she became even more perfect putting all her energies into her job and her family. Her husband was supportive and understanding. However he did experience great difficulty sexually as at times she would have no interest in sex and at other times be just the opposite. This caused some stress between them but when medication was mentioned, he, too, was opposed to it. Mrs. K. is now 50 years old and has not had a period in

nearly 2 years. During the past two years she had a
tremendous amount of energy and continues to take
Vitamins A E and B Complex daily. She's still experiencing hot flashes but their intensity and frequency
have decreased markedly. Her vagina muscles at times
become painful, then this symptom passes. "Intercourse is frequently painful these days," she states.
I asked her if she'd recommend cold turkey to anyone.
She replied that she wouldn't want to relive those
four years but is glad she hung in there.

Mrs. B. had been experiencing difficulty with
menopause for over a year. Frequent and very intense
hot flashes proved disruptive to her very outgoing
estrangement between her and her husband. A previously good sex life was by her own admission a disaster.
"I can't enjoy sex with Jack anymore, it's just too
painful. I feel like a dried up old prune. I'm
really afraid he's going to start seeing some younger
woman". When asked about estrogen replacement therapy
she replied that she wouldn't dare take it even though
her gynecologist had recommended it. When questioned
she indicated that her sister's physician was flatly
opposed to it. "I don't want cancer of the uterus,
and that's what you chance getting if you take those
hormones."

There are few instances of such diverse opinion
among medical doctors as that concerning the use of
estrogen replacement therapy. The idea is to replace
the hormone that a woman's ovaries have gradually
stopped producing during menopause. Many women will
testify to relief from symptoms such as hot flashes
and painful intercourse caused by vaginal dryness.
But some scientific studies have linked estrogen
supplements with the development of endometrial (uterine) cancer. Unfortunately there's no consensus of
opinion, within the medical profession. They're divid-
ed on what's called a risk-benefit problem.

However, there is agreement on the following.
First, before menopause, estrogen secreted in a
monthly cycle promotes cell growth or a thickening of
the lining of the uterus for a fertilized ovum (egg).
If conception does not occur then another hormone
called progesterone, causes a breakdown of this uterine lining resulting in menstruation. As the ovaries
wind down in their production of estrogen and pro-

gesterone during menopause other glands such as the adrenals take over producing smaller amounts of progesterone. This contributes to the premenstrual symptoms experienced by women in menopause. However, there's not enough progesterone to bring on a menstrual period. This may lead to hyperplasia, an overgrowth of the uterine lining (endometrium). Some doctors believe this to be a cause of uterine cancer.

One study involving over 1000 women from the Baltimore Maryland area concluded that estrogen replacement does increase a woman's chance of developing uterine cancer. But what was really significant was the relationship between the length of time using estrogen and uterine cancer. Women using estrogen for only a year or two had little risk but those with five or more years usage climbed to 17 times that of non-users.

Some popular articles on the subject would have us believe that you're playing Russian Roullette everytime you take the estrogen pill. But the incidence is very low. One woman in a thousand develops uterine cancer who has not taken estrogen and it's almost that low for those women who have been on estrogen for two to four years. It does however, increase to four to eight per thousand for those on estrogen replacement therapy for longer than four years. A recent publication in the New England Journal of Medicine states that researchers have concluded that giving women progesterone with estrogen reduces even further the possibility of uterine cancer. This certainly contradicts the highly publicized dangers of estrogen therapy. Unfortunately many women who could have been spared some of the discomforts of menopause by this therapy have been frightened away from it.

This is not a Carte Blanche endorsement of estrogen but rather a level headed approach to its possible use. If a woman has severe symptoms of menopause (usually one in three) she's a prospective candidate. However, if she has a previous history of breast cancer, has had a stroke, or blood clots or heart disease than she should avoid estrogen replacement therapy. Being cautious we should add those women who have taken DES (synthetic hormone) or whose mothers who took it while pregnant.

A once a year medical checkup for women on estrogen is recommended. These regular exams may detect any unusual symptoms such as vaginal bleeding. Close medical supervision further reduces the possibility of any problems developing whether from estrogen therapy or some other source.